Copyright ©2

QUINONES MD

Contents

Introduction 5

CBD 7

CBD vs. THC: What's the difference 7

What are the benefits of CBD 8

Is CBD legal 9

What does that mean for other CBD products 9

Buyer Beware 10

What Are the Risks of CBD Oil 12

Multiple Sclerosis 14

Types of Multiple Sclerosis 15

Four forms 15

Common category 16

Clinically isolated syndrome 16

Relapsing-remitting MS 17

Primary-progressive MS 18

Secondary-progressive MS 18

Symptoms 19

Disease course 21

Causes 22

Risk factors 22

Complications 23

Multiple Sclerosis Prognosis and Your Life Expectancy 24

Symptom progression and risk factors 26

Prognosis and complications 27

What can you expect 28

DIAGNOSIS 28

ACUTE THERAPY 32

DISEASE MODIFYING THERAPY 32

CONCLUSION 35

Mortality Trends in Patients With Multiple Sclerosis 36

Rates of survival increase over time 37

A second study parses MS data 38

New challenges for clinicians 39

Talking to Your Doctor About Changing MS Treatments 40

Your symptoms 40

Your lifestyle 41

Your reasons for wanting to switch medications 42

Tips for People Newly Diagnosed With Multiple Sclerosis 44

Ways to Cope With Your MS Diagnosis 45

CBD oil for mutiple sclerosis 52

Is it the Real Deal 54

What you Need to Know 56

Current Research on Cannabis and Multiple Sclerosis 57

The Role of CBD Products in Managing Multiple Sclerosis ... 58

Effects of Cannabinoids and CBD on Multiple Sclerosis 66

States That Have Approved Medical Cannabis for Multiple Sclerosis 67

Recent Studies on Cannabinoids and CBD's Effect on Multiple Sclerosis 69

CBD From Hemp and How It's Helped My MS 70

Hemp vs. marijuana 71

Quality issues 72

My experience 72

Strategies to Fine-Tune Your CBD Oil Dosage 76

Everyone Is Different 77

How Much CBD Oil Should I Take 78

Learn the Types of CBD Products 79

Choose a CBD Brand with a Dosage You Can Trust 82

Consider Why Your Health Would Benefit from CBD 83

Know You Cannot Overdose on CBD 85

Understand How Your Genetics Impact CBD Dosing 87

Rest Easy Knowing CBD Oil Is Not Physically Addictive 90

Get the Most Bang for Your Buck 91

Why is it so fascinating to the world of neurological disorders 92

Overcoming the stigma 92

Bottom line 94

Best CBD Oils for Multiple Sclerosis 94

Introduction

Multiple sclerosis (MS), the most common disabling neurologic disease of young people, afflicts approximately a quarter of a million Americans. The symptoms of MS result from recurrent attacks of inflammation in the central nervous system, which probably occur through an autoimmune mechanism. The target of the immune attack is myelin, the lipoprotein sheath that surrounds the axons and insulates them, and enhances nerve conduction. The white matter of the brain takes its name from the glistening white appearance of this lipid wrapping, which contains most of the pathways, tracts and axonal projections of the central nervous system. (The gray matter contains primarily the cell bodies of the neurons themselves.) Myelin is made by cells called oligodendrocytes and when it is inflamed and damaged, nerve conduction is disrupted and nerves thus lose function, thereby producing the neurologic symptoms of MS.

The cause of MS is unknown and its pathophysiology remains poorly understood. Patients are not born with MS, but rather some environmental factor apparently acts on genetically susceptible individuals to produce the disease; but the nature of that factor (such as whether or not it is a virus) remains elusive. The best accepted explanation postulates that macrophages present myelin antigens to appropriate T-cells, thereby activating the T-cells to proliferate. They then cross the blood-brain barrier through interactions with intercellular adhesion molecules and once inside the central nervous system, they release cytokines that further damage myelin and that perpetuate the immune response. The details of this process, including the nature of the triggering antigen, are still subject to speculation but there is strong evidence that MS is a T-cell mediated autoimmune attack on the central nervous system. Concomitant with the myelin destruction, there is also damage to the underlying axon, which leads to further disability.

Among the unanswered questions is whether MS is a single disease. It could be that different antigens are involved in different patients, different T-cells are activated, or the mechanisms of cell damage are different.

CBD

The cannabis plant contains more than 100 different chemical compounds known as cannabinoids, which interact with the body's endocannabinoid system in ways that researchers are still working toward understanding.

One of those cannabinoids is CBD, or cannabidiol (pronounced cann-a-bid-EYE-ol). CBD is non-psychoactive, which means it won't get you high — and there's a growing body of evidence that it has a number of health benefits.

CBD vs. THC: What's the difference

The main one is that CBD will not make you high. Of all those different cannabinoids found in the cannabis plant, the two best known are CBD and THC, or tetrahydrocannabinol.

CBD and THC are both found in marijuana, but it's the THC that's responsible for weed's mind-altering effects. THC is psychoactive; CBD is not. As long as your CBD products don't contain THC or contain very small amounts of it you can reap their potential benefits without going full Pineapple Express.

What are the benefits of CBD

There's plenty of anecdotal evidence that CBD helps treat a variety of ailments. People are turning to oils, gummies, and other CBD food and drink products to relax at the end of a long day. Retired NFL players are using CBD to manage physical pain, debilitating headaches, and sleeplessness. Spa clients are even using CBD skin products to fight signs of aging.

We're still in the early stages of understanding CBD's effects on the body, but there's already scientific evidence some of it funded by the U.S. government that CBD has legitimate medical benefits, too.

To name just a few: Animal research and small-scale human studies have pointed to CBD's anti-anxiety and anti-inflammatory properties, NPR reports. A study is underway to see how CBD helps patients with PTSD and alcohol use disorder, and another is exploring how CBD might help curb drug cravings in people with opioid addiction. Cannabinoids like CBD may also be effective at treating cancer-related side effects, according to the National Institutes of Health.

Is CBD legal

As of June 2018, the DEA still classified marijuana and its extracts — including CBD — as Schedule I substances, meaning CBD was banned by the feds. But when the FDA approved Epidiolex, the epilepsy medication that contains CBD, it initiated a 90-day window for the DEA to finally adjust its stance on cannabis.

In September, the DEA announced its decision: It would place Epidiolex in schedule 5 of the Controlled Substances Act the least restrictive classification. Some experts thought the DEA might reschedule CBD entirely, according to Business Insider. "DEA will continue to support sound and scientific research that promotes legitimate therapeutic uses for FDA-approved constituent components of cannabis, consistent with federal law," acting DEA administrator Uttam Dhillon said in a press release. "DEA is committed to continuing to work with our federal partners to seek ways to make the process for research more efficient and effective."

What does that mean for other CBD products

Unless it's Epidiolex, your CBD product is still classified as a Schedule I substance, which means it's banned by the feds. But as for state law, it depends on where you live and where your CBD came from: marijuana or hemp.

If your CBD comes from a plant that's legal in your state, then you're in the clear. (NORML has a helpful interactive map for cannabis laws by state.) The good news is, industrial hemp is legal nationwide — so if you want to be safe, choose a CBD product sourced from that.

Buyer Beware

It's the Wild West out there. Without any federal regulatory body checking labels, consumers have very little way of knowing what they're buying when they purchase CBD oil. Bonn-Miller co-authored a study that found that 26 percent of CBD products on the market contained less CBD than their label claimed. So the amount you need for an effective dose could vary drastically, not just from product to product, but from bottle to bottle of the same product.

"A CBD company may create a CBD oil, test it, and use the test results to create their label," Bonn-Miller says. "The problem is if they never test their product again, or they test it once a year, you have no idea whether each batch is the same as the first one that they used to create the label. The vast majority of companies are not using manufacturing standards that assure product consistency over time. Companies should be testing every batch they make and tossing batches that don't fall within the specs of their label."

As a consumer, you can look at the manufacturer's website to see whether they batch-test their products, or ask them directly. You could also send a sample of your CBD oil to a testing facility yourself, something Bonn-Miller says he would do if he were trying to treat someone with a severe issue such as epilepsy. Testing can also determine whether the product contains pesticides, heavy metals, or other toxins.

Bonn-Miller says in an ideal scenario, CBD companies would fund more of their own research to back up their claims.

"Right now, any claims and dosing recommendations by any company making a CBD product for the medical marijuana market is purely anecdotal," he says. "Asking 100 people who use your product whether they feel better isn't real science. The products on the market are also different from what was used in the scientific studies that they are basing their claims upon. If a study found an anti-anxiety effect when dosing humans with synthetic CBD, that doesn't mean that your CBD oil that contains 18 percent CBD is going to reduce anxiety. It might even have the opposite effect."

What Are the Risks of CBD Oil

The good news is that most of the official research done on CBD oil has shown that there are very few negative side effects from using it. However, CBD is not without some side effects. Most notably, in the clinical studies for epilepsy, sedation was one of the more common side effects. Decreased appetite and diarrhea were also seen in some patients. Depending on what other medicines they are taking, certain patients may need to have periodic blood tests to check on liver function.

In addition, CBD may cause some drug interactions. However, Bonn-Miller also adds that there is evidence that it does not have any dependence potential.

The legality of CBD is a real conundrum, which is a hurdle making it difficult for many necessary studies to get off the ground. Hemp (a cannabis plant with less than .3 percent THC) is legal in all 50 states, but when you start extracting CBD from the flowers of that plant, that might be technically redefining the plant as marijuana.

On the other hand, marijuana-derived CBD and anything else derived from a cannabis plant was still classified by the DEA as a Schedule I drug (defined as a drug with "no currently accepted medical use and a high potential for abuse") until October 2018. In 2016, the DEA stated that all extracts containing more than one cannabinoid would remain classified as Schedule I. However, the approval of

Epidiolex had an influence in changing this, and prescription CBD drugs with a THC content of below 0.1% have now been reclassified as Schedule 5, the lowest rating.

All this means that scientists can still only obtain marijuana-derived CBD from farms licensed by the National Institute on Drug Abuse (which until this year meant only one farm owned by the University of Mississippi). As for whether you should have a preference for CBD that comes from hemp, marijuana, or a pure synthetically produced version, there are some theories that THC—and even the smell and taste of cannabis— might make CBD more effective, but Bonn-Miller says these ideas have yet to be proven.

Then there's always the risk that you're wasting your money if some of the claims around CBD turn out to be overblown (or the product you're buying is bogus). But if CBD does even a fraction of what we think it does, by all means—pass the dropper on the left-hand side.

Multiple Sclerosis

Multiple sclerosis, or MS, is a long-lasting disease that can affect your brain, spinal cord, and the optic nerves in your eyes. It can cause problems with vision, balance, muscle control, and other basic body functions.

The effects are often different for everyone who has the disease. Some people have mild symptoms and don't need treatment. Others will have trouble getting around and doing daily tasks.

Multiple sclerosis (MS) is a potentially disabling disease of the brain and spinal cord (central nervous system).

In MS, the immune system attacks the protective sheath (myelin) that covers nerve fibers and causes communication problems between your brain and the rest of your body. Eventually, the disease can cause the nerves themselves to deteriorate or become permanently damaged.

Signs and symptoms of MS vary widely and depend on the amount of nerve damage and which nerves are affected. Some people with severe MS may lose the ability to walk independently or at all, while others may experience long periods of remission without any new symptoms.

There's no cure for multiple sclerosis. However, treatments can help speed recovery from attacks, modify the course of the disease and manage symptoms.

Types of Multiple Sclerosis

Multiple sclerosis (MS) is thought to be an autoimmune, inflammatory disease affecting the central nervous system and peripheral nerves.

The cause remains unknown, but some studies indicate a link between the Epstein Barr Virus, while others indicate environmental factors, a lack of vitamin D, or parasites as a stimulus of the persistent immune response in the central nervous system. It can be unpredictable and, in some cases, disabling. But not all forms of MS are the same.

To help distinguish between the different types of the condition, the National Multiple Sclerosis Society (NMSS) identified four distinct categories.

Four forms

To accurately define the different forms of MS, in 1996, the NMSS surveyed a group of scientists who specialized in MS patient care and research. After analyzing the scientists' responses, the organization categorized the condition into four primary types.

These course definitions were updated in 2013 to reflect advances in research. They are:

- clinically isolated syndrome (CIS)
- relapsing-remitting MS (RRMS)
- primary-progressive MS (PPMS)
- secondary-progressive MS (SPMS)

Common category

The four categories defined by the NMSS are now relied upon by the medical community at large and create a common language for diagnosing and treating MS. The categories' classifications are based on how far the disease has progressed in each patient.

Clinically isolated syndrome

Clinically isolated syndrome (CIS) is a single episode of neurologic symptoms that lasts 24 hours or more. Your symptoms cannot be tied to fever, infection, or other illness. They're the result of inflammation or demyelination in the central nervous system.

You might have only one symptom (monofocal episode) or several (multifocal episode). If you have CIS, you may never experience another episode. Or this episode could be your first MS attack. If an MRI detects brain lesions similar to those found in people with MS, there's a 60 to

80 percent chance you'll have another episode and a diagnosis of MS within a few years.

At this time, you might have a diagnosis of MS if an MRI detects older lesions in a different part of your central nervous system. That would mean you've had a previous attack, even if you weren't aware of it. Your doctor might also diagnose MS if your cerebrospinal fluid contains oligoclonal bands.

Relapsing-remitting MS

The most common type is relapsing-remitting MS (RRMS). According to the NMSS, approximately 85 percent of people with MS have this type at the time of diagnosis.

When you have RRMS you may experience:

- clearly defined relapses or flare-ups that result in episodes of intensive worsening of your neurologic function
- partial or complete remissions or recovery periods after the relapses and between attacks when the disease stops progressing
- mild to severe symptoms as well as relapses and remissions that last for days or months

- Progressive types of MS
- While the vast majority of people with MS have the RRMS form, some are diagnosed with a progressive form of the disease: primary-progressive MS (PPMS) or secondary-progressive MS (SPMS).
- Each of these types indicates that the disease continues to worsen without improvement.

Primary-progressive MS

This form of MS progresses slowly yet steadily from the time of its onset. Symptoms stay at the same level of intensity without decreasing, and there are no remission periods. In essence, patients with PPMS experience a fairly continuous worsening of their condition.

However, there can be variations in the rate of progression over the course of the disease — as well as the possibility of minor improvements (usually temporary) and occasional plateaus in symptom progression.

The NMSS estimates that approximately 15 percent of people with MS have PPMS at the onset of the condition.

Secondary-progressive MS

SPMS is more of a mixed bag. Initially, it may involve a period of relapsing-remitting activity, with symptom flare-ups followed by recovery periods. Yet the disability of MS doesn't disappear between cycles.

Instead, this period of fluctuation is followed by a steady worsening of the condition. People with SPMS may experience minor remissions or plateaus in their symptoms, but this isn't always the case.

Without treatment, about half of people with RRMS go on to develop SPMS within a decade.

Type casting

Early MS can be challenging for doctors to diagnose. As such, it can be helpful to understand the characteristics and symptoms of MS at the time of initial diagnosis — particularly since the vast majority of people with the disease exhibit characteristics of relapsing-remitting MS.

Although MS currently has no cure, it isn't normally fatal. In fact, most people who have MS never become severely disabled, according to the NMSS.

Identifying MS early at the relapsing-remitting stage can help ensure prompt treatment to avoid developing more progressive forms of the illness.

Symptoms
- MS-related nervous system damage

- Myelin damage and the nervous system
- Multiple sclerosis signs and symptoms may differ greatly from person to person and over the course of the disease depending on the location of affected nerve fibers. They may include:
- Numbness or weakness in one or more limbs that typically occurs on one side of your body at a time, or the legs and trunk
- Partial or complete loss of vision, usually in one eye at a time, often with pain during eye movement
- Prolonged double vision
- Tingling or pain in parts of your body
- Electric-shock sensations that occur with certain neck movements, especially bending the neck forward (Lhermitte sign)
- Tremor, lack of coordination or unsteady gait
- Slurred speech
- Fatigue
- Dizziness
- Problems with bowel and bladder function
- When to see a doctor

See a doctor if you experience any of the above symptoms for unknown reasons.

Disease course

Most people with MS have a relapsing-remitting disease course. They experience periods of new symptoms or relapses that develop over days or weeks and usually improve partially or completely. These relapses are followed by quiet periods of disease remission that can last months or even years.

Small increases in body temperature can temporarily worsen signs and symptoms of MS, but these aren't considered disease relapses.

About 60 to 70 percent of people with relapsing-remitting MS eventually develop a steady progression of symptoms, with or without periods of remission, known as secondary-progressive MS.

The worsening of symptoms usually includes problems with mobility and gait. The rate of disease progression varies greatly among people with secondary-progressive MS.

Some people with MS experience a gradual onset and steady progression of signs and symptoms without any relapses. This is known as primary-progressive MS.

Causes

The cause of multiple sclerosis is unknown. It's considered an autoimmune disease in which the body's immune system attacks its own tissues. In the case of MS, this immune system malfunction destroys myelin (the fatty substance that coats and protects nerve fibers in the brain and spinal cord).

Myelin can be compared to the insulation coating on electrical wires. When the protective myelin is damaged and nerve fiber is exposed, the messages that travel along that nerve may be slowed or blocked. The nerve may also become damaged itself.

It isn't clear why MS develops in some people and not others. A combination of genetics and environmental factors appears to be responsible.

Risk factors

- These factors may increase your risk of developing multiple sclerosis:
- Age. MS can occur at any age, but most commonly affects people between the ages of 15 and 60.
- Sex. Women are about twice as likely as men are to develop MS.

- Family history. If one of your parents or siblings has had MS, you are at higher risk of developing the disease.
- Certain infections. A variety of viruses have been linked to MS, including Epstein-Barr, the virus that causes infectious mononucleosis.
- Race. White people, particularly those of Northern European descent, are at highest risk of developing MS. People of Asian, African or Native American descent have the lowest risk.
- Climate. MS is far more common in countries with temperate climates, including Canada, the northern United States, New Zealand, southeastern Australia and Europe.
- Certain autoimmune diseases. You have a slightly higher risk of developing MS if you have thyroid disease, type 1 diabetes or inflammatory bowel disease.
- Smoking. Smokers who experience an initial event of symptoms that may signal MS are more likely than nonsmokers to develop a second event that confirms relapsing-remitting MS.

Complications

People with multiple sclerosis also may develop:

- Muscle stiffness or spasms
- Paralysis, typically in the legs

- Problems with bladder, bowel or sexual function
- Mental changes, such as forgetfulness or mood swings
- Depression
- Epilepsy

Multiple Sclerosis Prognosis and Your Life Expectancy

PROGNOSIS

Multiple sclerosis is seldom fatal and life expectancy is shortened by only a few months. Concerns about prognosis center primarily on the quality of life and prospects for disability. Most patients and physicians harbor an unfounded view of MS as a relentlessly progressive, inevitably disabling disease. The truth is that 15 years after the onset of MS, only about 20% of patients are bedridden or institutionalized. Another 20% may require a wheelchair, or use crutches, or a cane to ambulate, but fully 60% will be ambulatory without assistance and some will have little deficit at all. Perhaps as many as 1/3 of all patients with MS go through life without any persistent disability, and suffer only intermittent, transient episodes of symptoms.

When it comes to the prognosis for multiple sclerosis (MS), there's both good news and bad news. Although no known cure exists for MS, there is some good news about life expectancy. Because MS isn't a fatal disease, people who have MS essentially have the same life expectancy as the general population.

A closer look at prognosis

According to the National Multiple Sclerosis Society (NMSS), the majority of people who have MS will experience a relatively normal life span. On average, most people with MS live about seven years less than the general population. Those with MS tend to die from many of the same conditions, such as cancer and heart disease, as people who don't have the condition. Apart from cases of severe MS, which are rare, the prognosis for longevity is generally good.

However, people who have MS also have to contend with other issues that can decrease their quality of life. Even though most will never become severely disabled, many experience symptoms that cause pain, discomfort, and inconvenience.

Another way of evaluating the prognosis for MS is to examine how disabilities resulting from the condition's symptoms may affect people. According to the NMSS, around two-thirds of people with MS are able to walk without a wheelchair two decades after their diagnosis. Some people will need crutches or a cane to remain ambulatory. Others use an electric scooter or wheelchair to help them cope with fatigue or balance difficulties.

Symptom progression and risk factors

It's hard to predict how MS will progress in every person. The severity of the disease varies widely from person to person.

Around 45 percent of those with MS aren't severely affected by the disease.

Most people living with MS will undergo a certain amount of disease progression.

To help determine your personal prognosis, it helps to understand the risk factors that may indicate a greater chance of developing a severe form of the condition. According to the Mayo Clinic, women are twice as likely as men to develop MS. Additionally, certain factors indicate a higher risk for more severe symptoms, including the following:

- You're over 40 at the initial onset of symptoms.
- Your initial symptoms affect many parts of your body.

- Your initial symptoms affect mental functioning, urinary control, or motor control.

Prognosis and complications

Prognosis is affected by the type of MS. Primary progressive MS (PPMS) is characterized by a steady decline in function without relapses or remissions. There may be some periods of inactive decline as every case is different. However, the steady progression continues.

For the relapsing forms of MS, there are several guidelines that may help predict prognosis. People with MS tend to do better if they experience:

- few symptom attacks in the initial few years post-diagnosis
- a longer amount of time passing between attacks
- a complete recovery from their attacks
- symptoms related to sensory problems, such as tingling, vision loss, or numbness
- neurological exams that appear almost normal five years after diagnosis

While most people with MS have a close-to-normal life expectancy, it can be difficult for doctors to predict whether their condition will worsen or improve, since the disease varies so much from person to person. In most cases, however, MS isn't a fatal condition.

What can you expect

MS generally affects quality of life more than longevity. While certain rare types of MS can potentially affect lifespan, they are the exception rather than the rule. People with MS must contend with many difficult symptoms that will affect their lifestyle, but they can rest assured that their life expectancy essentially mirrors that of people who don't have the condition.

DIAGNOSIS

MS can be among the most difficult of all diseases to diagnose because of the bewildering number of symptoms it causes and the multiple ways in which they can present. The "typical" MS patient is a young woman with abrupt, focal neurologic symptoms occurring discretely or in combinations, lasting weeks to months and then resolving, with new or recur-rent symptoms developing months to years later. The diagnosis may be especially difficult, or indeed impossible, when the patient is older, when symptoms are strictly progressive, or when there has been only one episode of neurologic dysfunction. Tests can buttress the clinical diagnosis of MS, but no laboratory findings are pathognomonic and all tests have pitfalls that limit their usefulness.

Magnetic resonance imaging (MRI) is a very sensitive but disappointingly non-specific technique for visualizing the inflammatory lesions of MS, which appear as multiple, irregular, confluent areas of increased signal intensity within the white matter of the brain, particularly around the ventricles. Nearly 90% of patients with MS have abnormal MRI scans. Various analyses and algorithms have shown that an MRI of the head should be the first test ordered to evaluate suspected MS patients. The major disadvantage of MRI remains its lack of specificity, since many conditions mimic MS on MRI. Too frequently, these "false positives" often inappropriately label patients with the diagnosis of MS and over-diagnosis of MS based on MRI changes.

Abnormalities in the cerebrospinal fluid (CSF) are sufficiently common and characteristic to make CSF analysis fairly accurate for the diagnosis of MS. Spinal fluid protein and white blood cell counts are occasionally mildly elevated, but the most useful findings are the increases in the immunoglobulin G (IgG) level and synthesis rate. Immunoglobulins in the spinal fluid, presumably reflecting the underlying autoimmune activation, appear as distinct oligoclonal bands on CSF electrophoresis. The pattern formed by these bands varies from patient to patient, but they are present in some form in approximately 90% of all MS patients, while the few other diseases that produce similar banding are seldom mistaken for MS. The major obstacle to the use of CSF for the diagnosis of MS is the reluctance of patients to undergo lumbar puncture.

Evoked potentials play a more limited role in diagnosing MS. Evoked potentials measure conduction along specific central nervous system pathways by recording the electroencephalographic response to visual, auditory, or sensory stimulation.

A slowing in conduction is presumed to reflect inflammation and demyelination in that pathway, thus detecting an asymptomatic MS lesion. The sensitivity and specificity of evoked potentials do not approach those of the MRI or CSF but they sometimes uncover unsuspected lesions and thereby heighten the probability of MS.

The list of medical conditions that can cause multi-focal neurologic problems in young people is quite extensive and so the differential diagnosis of MS is far ranging. Table 3 is a non-exhaustive list of some of the more common conditions that mimic MS.

Traditionally, the diagnosis of MS depends upon showing that there is sclerosis (scarring or inflammation) that is multiple—patients must have two separate CNS lesions that have occurred in two or more separate episodes, which is to say they must have lesions disseminated in space and in time. These must cause white matter symptoms not gray matter symptoms. The neurological examination should show these objective abnormalities (preferably in a young patient between the ages of 20 and 40). Importantly, there should be no other disease accounting for the symptoms. In addition to these clinical criteria, the diagnosis can be supported using laboratory testing such as MRI scans, CSF analysis and evoked potentials. There nevertheless remain many pitfalls and nuances in the diagnosis of MS, and ultimately physicians often rely on their own judgment to diagnose MS rather than relying on predetermined or "official" criteria.4

Many patients who suffer an isolated monosymptomatic episode of demyelination, such as optic neuritis or transverse myelitis, will ultimately develop a second inflammatory event and so will be diagnosed as having MS. This is particularly true if MRI scanning of the brain at the time of their initial demyelinating event reveals white matter changes characteristic of MS. Therefore, patients with a single episode of demyelination and abnormal MRI scan of the brain are often presumed to be suffering from MS already. (This is true even though most "official" diagnostic criteria would not classify these patients as definite MS.) There remain some cases of clinically isolated syndromes with normal head MRI's who apparently never develop clinically definite MS.

ACUTE THERAPY

Acute relapses of MS are usually treated with corticosteroids. There are few good controlled studies of the effectiveness of steroids, the optimum dosage, route of administration, duration of treatment, or most appropriate indications for their use. Nevertheless, steroid treatments have become a traditional and accepted standard of practice for new attacks of MS and there is a universal sense that they shorten symptoms, enhance well-being and provide many benefits for acute relapses. A standard regimen uses intravenous methylprednisolone (Solumedrol) 1 gram daily for three to five days, sometimes (but not always, depending on physician preference) followed by a tapering dose of oral steroids. Steroids reduce inflammation, seal the blood/brain barrier, enhance nerve conduction and alter the immune system, all of which are potentially beneficial in treating MS. Whatever benefits they have seem to be limited primarily to acute attacks and it is less clear that they can fundamentally alter the natural history of MS or prevent ultimate disability.

DISEASE MODIFYING THERAPY

Five drugs are currently approved by the Food and Drug Administration as disease modifying agents that alter the natural history of relapsing-remitting MS. The four self-administered drugs are intramuscular beta-interferon-la (Avonex), subcutaneous beta-interferon-la (Rebif), subcutaneous betainterferon-lb (Betaseron), and glatiramer acetate (Copaxone). These medications all reduce the number of attacks in relapsing-remitting MS. They seem to have little effect once the disease has entered a secondary progressive phase. The mechanism of action of these drugs is unknown, but the interferons probably induce secretion of a variety of immunomodulatory proteins while glatiramer probably inhibits the activation of myelin reactive T-cells.5

Avonex is a preparation of recombinant human beta-interferon-la, administered in a dosage of 6 million IU intramuscularly once a week. Rebif is an identical preparation, administered as 12 million IU subcutaneously three times a week. Betaseron is recombinant beta-interferon-lb, which differs from Avonex and Rebif only in some minor alterations of a single amino acid substitution and less glycosolation, though it is doubtful that these changes make it truly a different drug. It is given as 12 million IU subcutaneously every other day. Copaxone differs from all these drugs because it is not an interferon but rather is a synthetic polypeptide composed of sequences of four amino acids that share many antigenic similarities to myelin basic protein and appears to alter the immune response to myelin. It is a subcutaneous preparation given daily. There are still no definitive head-to-head comparisons of these drugs and so the differences among them (such as whether higher doses of interferons confer greater benefits) are still a matter of conjecture and debate. At present, these four drugs can be considered approximately equal in efficacy and therapeutic decisions are often made based on convenience of dosage, route of administration, side effects, concern for neutralizing antibodies (which develop against the interferons after about a year in 2 to 30% of patients) and similar practical issues. Although these medications have some benefits in minimizing the rate of attacks, it is not known whether they will delay the accumulation of neurologic deficits and so postpone disability. Their long-term benefits are thus unclear.6

For secondary progressive MS, the most convincing data favors mitoxantrone (Novantrone) as most likely to retard progression and delay disability. Novantrone is a well-established cancer chemotherapeutic drug, primarily effective for lymphomas and leukemias, with broad immune-altering properties. It can delay the accumulation of disability in patients with secondary progressive MS when administered in a dosage of, 12 mg/m2 intravenously every three months. Such periodic treatments can slow the progression of MS but, when a cumulative dose of 100–140 mg/m2 has been given, the risk of irreversible toxicity from the drug precludes further administration. The primary toxicity is myocardial damage, and so echocardiograms and ejection fractions are followed periodically throughout treatment. For most patients, toxicity limits treatment to a duration of only two or three years and so Novantrone should be considered a short-term treatment option.

CONCLUSION

In just the past few years, research has further clarified the cellular and molecular events that accompany an MS immune attack on myelin and has raised speculation that there could be several diseases comprising what we now call MS. Epidemiological studies have also clarified the prognosis and reaffirmed that many patients do well. The distinction between relapsing-remitting MS and secondary progressive MS has assumed increasing importance, in part because of different responses to treatment. New criteria for the diagnosis of MS have also been developed to take advantage of the extraordinary sensitivity of MR imaging. Most importantly, in less than 10 years, five new drugs have been developed with proven ability to alter the natural history of MS and mitigate the disease. These advances have completely altered the clinician's approach to the patient with MS and foreshadow new hope for the ultimate conquest of this disease.

Mortality Trends in Patients With Multiple Sclerosis

Data from a number of large registries indicate that people with multiple sclerosis (MS) have a life expectancy 7 to 14 years less than that of the general population.1 Less is known, however, about the causes of death among people with MS or trends in mortality over time.2 Two recent studies conducted in Northern Europe shed new light on these issues.2,3 In a Swedish study, Burkill and colleagues evaluated trends in mortality and causes of death among patients with MS.2 In a Danish study, Koch-Henriksen and colleagues assessed short-term all-cause mortality among patients with MS to determine whether it has changed in roughly the last 50 years.3

The Burkill study identified people diagnosed with MS in Sweden between 1964 and 2012, based on nationwide registry data. Patients with MS (29,617) were matched with controls who didn't have MS (296,164) in a 1:10 ratio. Causes of death were identified using a corresponding Swedish registry.2

Take Note

The life expectancy of people with multiple sclerosis (MS) is 7 to 14 years less than that of the general population.

Although the reason is unclear, a pair of new studies finds that mortality has decreased over time in people with MS.

While these changes are promising, clinicians may face special challenges as MS of longer duration is superimposed on normal aging.

Rates of survival increase over time

Using Cox proportional hazard models, the study found that people with MS were at greater risk of death from any cause compared to controls (hazard ratio [HR] 2.92, 95% confidence interval [CI] 2.86 to 2.99). The greatest differences between the 2 groups were in death due to respiratory conditions (HR 5.07, 95% CI 4.87 to 5.26) and death due to infectious diseases (HR 4.07, 95% CI 3.70 to 4.47), often sepsis.

These findings, however, were for the entire study period; when the period 1968 to 1980 was compared to the period 2001 to 2012, a significant decrease in mortality was found among patients with MS, both overall and for each specific cause of death evaluated. (In addition to respiratory and infectious diseases, these causes of death included accidents, suicides, and cardiovascular diseases.) In particular, the hazard ratio decreased from 6.52 (95% CI 5.79 to 7.34) in 1968 to 1980 to 2.08 (95% CI 1.95 to 2.22) in 2001 to 2012.

"The findings highlight notable improvements in survival among MS patients over time," says Sarah Burkill, MSc, a doctoral candidate at the Karolinska Institute in Stockholm and lead author of the study. "However, longevity remains shorter compared with the general population."

"While the changes in survival are promising, more progress in the care of MS patients is required to reduce mortality further," Burkill added.

A second study parses MS data

Koch-Henriksen and colleagues identified people with MS from the Danish MS Registry, including those with onset of definite or probable MS from 1950 through 1999.3 By searching additional national databases, they "followed patients from onset until death, emigration, or end of follow-up in 2015, whichever came first," and calculated population mortality (expected numbers of deaths).3

Using these data, the researchers determined the excess number of deaths per 1000 person-years, also known as the excess death rate (EDR), as well as the standardized mortality ratio (SMR) of observed to expected deaths. When analyzing mortality trends, the team divided the participants into 5, 10-year onset cohorts beginning with 1950, 1960, 1970, 1980, and 1990, and they included only the first 15 years after onset of MS, to ensure that everyone in the study would be followed for the same amount of time.

Among 18,847 people with MS included in the analysis, the study reported 6102 actual deaths, with only 2492 of them expected. Koch-Henriksen and colleagues calculated an EDR of 10.63 (95% CI 10.19 to 11.09) and an SMR of 2.45 (95% CI 2.39 to 2.51). They determined that the 15-year EDR decreased over time from 11.29 (95% CI 9.95 to 12.73) in the 1950 to 1959 onset cohort to 2.56 (95% CI 1.98 to 3.18) in the 1990 to 1999 onset cohort. Moreover, SMR dropped from 4.48 (95% CI 4.06 to 4.92) to 1.80 (95% CI 1.62 to 1.99).

New challenges for clinicians

"Decrease in excess mortality is encouraging, particularly if it's associated with longer time to irreversible disability," says lead study author Nils Koch-Henriksen, MD, DMSci, of the Danish MS Registry in Copenhagen and the Department of Clinical Epidemiology at the University of Aarhus in Denmark. While Dr. Koch-Henriksen could offer no definitive explanation for the observed decrease in mortality, he notes that the prevalence of MS is likely to increase in the coming years, if only because people with MS are living longer.

"Clinicians will see more patients with MS of longer disease duration and at higher ages, and thereby with increased risk of age-related comorbidities," says Dr. Koch-Henriksen. "Clinicians may also meet special challenges when MS is combined with normal aging."

Talking to Your Doctor About Changing MS Treatments

Multiple sclerosis (MS) is a complex and individual disease. Each person experiences it differently. When it comes to treatment, no two people have the same results. Some treatments may work well for you, but others may not. If you're not satisfied with your current treatment, you might want to try something else.

There are many reasons to consider changing treatments. Your current medication might have side effects that bother you, or it may no longer seem to be as effective as it was. Here are some topics to discuss with your doctor if you're considering switching to a new MS treatment.

Your symptoms

MS can cause many symptoms that vary in frequency and severity, even when your treatment is effective in preventing progression or new lesions. This can happen because symptom management and disease management are two different things. You might not be feeling well, but that doesn't mean your treatment is no longer working, and vice versa.

Speak to your doctor about your symptoms and how you can manage them. Research shows that managing symptoms is important for maintaining better quality of life. Your doctor can prescribe disease-modifying therapies (DMTs) and other medications and therapies to help manage your symptoms.

Some common MS-related symptoms include:

- pain
- spasticity (muscle stiffness)
- bladder issues

When your symptoms are under control, you can continue with an effective disease management treatment.

Your lifestyle

When you choose an MS treatment, how it will affect your lifestyle may be a big consideration. Your doctor will understand that. It's important to find a treatment that will keep you feeling your best while allowing you to live normally.

You need to take MS treatments on a long-term basis for them to be successful. When you start to consider your options, ask your doctor some questions about how the treatment may affect your lifestyle. These could include:

- How often will I need to take this medication?
- How easy is it to administer?
- What are the side effects I can most likely expect?
- What impact will other medications have on my lifestyle?
- Will I need any special monitoring or tests?
- What are the risks of taking other medications with this treatment?

All medications carry some sort of risk of complication. You should factor the risks into your decision. Your doctor can help you weigh these risks against the benefits. But you'll ultimately be responsible for making the final decision about your treatment.

Your reasons for wanting to switch medications

There are reasons you're on your current treatment. Before switching medications, your doctor will want to know why you want to make a change.

You'll want to discuss how your current treatment is making you feel both physically and emotionally, including:

- troubling side effects
- concerns that treatment is no longer working
- concerns about the cost of treatment
- difficulties taking or injecting your medication
- issues with dosing or remembering to take your medication

Rather than switching treatments, your doctor may be able to offer other solutions to make your current treatment work for you. This could include:

- modifying your dose
- prescribing a more affordable generic version
- giving you a planned break from your treatment

Before you think about switching treatments, make sure that you've been taking your current medication properly. Not taking medication as prescribed is one of the most common causes of poor response to treatment.

Any new changes to your diet, or other medications you take, may also affect the way your MS treatment works. Be sure to tell your doctor if you're doing anything differently or taking new medications for other conditions.

The takeaway

There are many things to consider before beginning any treatment for MS. It's also necessary to think about why switching to another MS treatment might be more beneficial.

Make your choices about treatment options easier by talking with your doctor. And make the discussion as productive as possible by asking questions. You need the answers to make an informed decision about the best treatment for you.

Tips for People Newly Diagnosed With Multiple Sclerosis

- Starting treatment early can slow the progression of MS.
- No two people have exactly the same MS symptoms.
- Both conventional and complementary therapies can help to ease MS symptoms.

A multiple sclerosis diagnosis can be frightening and overwhelming, but while you may feel very much alone, you are by no means the only one dealing with this condition.

Multiple sclerosis is the most common neurological disease in young adults, usually striking between ages 20 and 40. An estimated 400,000 people in the United States and 2.3 million people worldwide have MS — and there's one new U.S. diagnosis of MS every hour, according to the National Multiple Sclerosis Society (NMSS). The good news: MS symptoms can usually be managed successfully.

"Having MS today is much different from what it was in the past, because we now have a number of new and promising treatments that do a good job at controlling symptoms," says William Sheremata, MD, professor emeritus of clinical neurology at the University of Miami's Miller School of Medicine in Florida.

Ways to Cope With Your MS Diagnosis

If you're newly diagnosed with MS, these tips can help you manage the disease.

1. Learn as much as possible about MS. There are many myths and misconceptions about multiple sclerosis, and without the facts, your MS diagnosis can be scarier than necessary.

MS is a chronic inflammatory disease affecting the central nervous system. It is thought to be caused by the immune system attacking myelin, the protective insulation covering nerve fibers in the brain and spinal cord. Myelin is destroyed and replaced by scars of hardened tissue (lesions), and some underlying nerves are damaged, causing a broad range of symptoms.

But MS is almost never fatal, and it is possible to live a fulfilling life with the disease. Your doctor and organizations like the NMSS can help you understand more about MS and stay up-to-date on new treatments.

2. Be sure your MS diagnosis is definitive. MS is not an easy disease to diagnose, so getting a definitive diagnosis can take some time. Various tests may be used to make a diagnosis, including magnetic resonance imaging (MRI), evoked potentials (EP), and spinal fluid analysis (spinal tap), as well as a neurological exam. According to the latest criteria, your physician must do all the following to make an MS diagnosis:

Find evidence of damage in two separate areas of the central nervous system

Find evidence that the incidents of damage occurred at least one month apart

Rule out all other possible diseases and diagnoses

For many people, getting a definitive diagnosis is actually a relief — because they now have a name for unexplained symptoms.

3. Understand that MS symptoms are unpredictable. No two people have exactly the same MS symptoms, and you may have different symptoms from time to time. MS symptoms can include numbness, blurred vision, loss of balance, poor coordination, slurred speech, tremors, extreme fatigue, problems with memory, bladder dysfunction, paralysis, blindness, and more. But these symptoms are unpredictable.

"Over the course of the disease, some MS symptoms will come and go, while others may be long lasting," Dr. Sheremata says. "It will be different for each MS patient."

4. Don't delay MS treatment. After receiving an MS diagnosis, it's important to start treatment as soon as possible. A number of FDA-approved medications have been shown to lessen the frequency and severity of MS attacks, or relapses, as well as to slow the progression of MS.

"The disease is more likely to progress and possibly lead to disability if you don't begin treatment early in the disease," Sheremata says.

5. Track your MS symptoms. Keeping a record of your MS symptoms and how you are feeling will help your doctor determine how the disease is progressing and whether the medications you are taking are working. It will also help you and your doctor recognize a relapse, which is characterized by a worsening of previous symptoms or the appearance of a new symptom that lasts more than 24 hours.

If you're having symptoms that you think are related to MS, write them down in a log. Include when the symptom happened, details of what it felt like, and how long it lasted.

6. Avoid MS symptom triggers. Extreme fatigue is a common indicator of an impending relapse, which can last for days, weeks, or months. But certain triggers are thought to bring on relapses or make them worse. Stress, lack of sleep, infection, and hot baths or anything else that can lead to overheating can cause a worsening of MS symptoms and may even trigger a relapse.

In some cases, a worsening of symptoms may actually be a pseudo-relapse, in which the symptoms resolve quickly as the body cools down or a minor infection clears up.

Drinking alcohol in excess is discouraged for people with MS because intoxication causes poor coordination and slurred speech, which can compound existing MS symptoms.

7. Find the right doctor for you. MS is a lifelong disease, so it's important to be under the care of an MS specialist who is a good match for you. The neurologist who provided your initial MS diagnosis may not be the specialist you want to stick with for life. The NMSS Partners in MS Care program can help you locate neurologists in your area (within the United States) with expertise in treating MS. Support groups for people with MS (available through hospitals and the NMSS) are also helpful for getting doctor referrals.

8. Consider complementary and alternative medicine. In addition to taking medication to control your MS symptoms, you may want to consider complementary treatments, such as biofeedback, acupuncture, guided imagery, meditation, massage, tai chi, yoga, and dietary

supplements. The majority of people with MS turn to these and other forms of complementary medicine to relieve symptoms, according to the NMSS. Such natural therapies are often used for pain relief, fatigue, and stress.

9. Think about whom you'll tell. Announcing to your employer that you have MS could negatively affect your job security, employment options, and career path. Before disclosing the disease at your workplace, learn about your rights under the Americans with Disabilities Act.

Of course, you'll want to tell your closest family members and friends, particularly those who know you well enough to notice that something is wrong. But you are not obligated to share news of your MS diagnosis with everyone in your life. Instead, pick the people who will be most supportive and helpful as you learn to live with the disease.

10. Don't give up hope. Although there currently is no cure for MS, newer treatments can slow the progression of the disease, improving your quality of life and preventing disability. And research is ongoing, with the goal of developing even better treatments in the near future that

will stop progression and even restore functions and abilities that have been lost.

CBD oil for mutiple sclerosis

Several studies have demonstrated the therapeutic potential of cannabis and its derivate products to manage the symptoms of multiple sclerosis (MS) and other neurodegenerative diseases. But there is still much to be done to enhance their use and accessibility to patients who may benefit from these therapies, according to a recent presentation by Matthew Makelky, PharmD.

The use of marijuana for medical purposes is currently legal in 29 states in the U.S. Only nine of those states also allow recreational marijuana use. With the trend toward legalizing cannabis, additional pressure lies on clinicians who prescribe it to ensure proper use and administration.

Cannabis contains more than 100 pharmacologically active compounds (cannabinoids), with the most studied compounds being the tetrahydrocannabinol (THC) and cannabidiol (CBD). Both have been evaluated for their potential to modulate spasticity associated with MS, as well as to manage seizures, inflammation, pain, anxiety, and other conditions.

Theoretically, CBD holds greater therapeutic potential than THC, since the first does not have the psychoactive properties that accompany THC use. Still, this compound is linked to some adverse side effects, such as drowsiness, decreased appetite, diarrhea, fatigue, and convulsion.

The THC compound is the one responsible for the "high" experience people feel when consuming cannabis, and is linked to increased neurological risk. THC has been associated with altered brain development and cognitive impairment when used in early adolescence, but also to an increased risk of chronic psychosis disorders.

According to the American Academy of Neurology, the use of oral cannabis extract (OCE) and synthetic THC improved spasticity-related symptoms and pain in patients with MS.

n contrast, AAN considers there is limited or insufficient evidence demonstrating the effectiveness of oromucosal cannabinoid spray, such as Sativex (nabiximols), or smoked cannabis for these indications.

As for treating MS-related urinary symptoms and tremor, none of the tested forms of cannabinoids have shown compelling evidence of effectiveness, according to Makelky.

There are some cannabinoid-based drugs already available on the market and others are under development. Because of the different effects of each cannabinoid compound, finding suitable dosages and methods of administration, as well as optimal frequency of use, may be both challenging and risky.

Also, cannabinoids may chemically react with other prescribed drugs — increasing or reducing their effects — which adds another layer of potential hazard that should be discussed between patients and clinicians.

In summary, cannabis-derived compounds hold potential to treat MS and "to help specific disease states," Makelky said. Still, there is a lot to learn about "the complex metabolism and interaction profiles" of these compounds, he added.

Is it the Real Deal

What's so impossibly frustrating about the lack of attention and research CBD gets as a viable multiple sclerosis treatment is the fact that, as we said, the U.S. government holds a patent on the drug for its medically-proven ability to limit neurological damage.

This simple fact can be considered in one of two ways. On the one hand, the notion that the cannabinoid is recognized by the National Institute of Health as a neuroprotectant is virtually a signed, sealed, and delivered acknowledgment of its ability to treat multiple sclerosis.

On the other, more sinister hand, the fact that the drug is owned by the federal government means it's highly unlikely it'll ever get into the hands of Big Pharma.

Superficially this might seem like a really good thing, but at the end of the day all it means is that 'conventional' physicians and medical professionals will never recognize it as a truly viable multiple sclerosis treatment. Rather, they'll continue to push the risky, insanely expensive pharmaceutical drugs which are backed by FDA research and regulations.

| "Will the U.S. Government's patent limit the likelihood that CBD gets approved as a multiple sclerosis treatment?"

At the end of the day, due to its all-powerful financial hand, Big Pharma will likely have the final say in terms of what's going to be available in terms of treatment, and what's not. The fact that CBD oil for multiple sclerosis has shown potential to be an efficient and productive form of medication for the disease is irrelevant – if it's not financially viable for the drug manufacturers, you're not going to see the majority of physicians prescribing it.

And of course, there's nothing financially viable about a 100% natural plant that you can grow in your own home.

What you Need to Know

One thing we didn't necessarily clarify is the difference in function between CBD and THC. THC, of course, is the archetypal marijuana component; it's what's responsible for getting us high, and is what has been the driving force behind generations of legal condemnation and "lazy stoner" typecasts.

CBD, on the other hand, has none of these psychoactive properties – it won't get you any more 'high' than a tablet of ibuprofen will.

Rather, the molecule functions as an "endocannabinoid supplement"; that is to say, our bodies are chock-full of 100% natural cannabinoid receptors that work hand-in-hand with 100% naturally endocannabinoids – if there is an absence or deficiency in the production of these endocannabinoids, the receptors will not be able to function properly. And it just so happens that the central nervous system is the region of the body that's most densely populated with cannabinoid receptors – the same region where multiple sclerosis attacks nerve fibers.

Could, then, multiple sclerosis potentially be a disease hinged on a basic endocannabinoid deficiency? While no one can answer that question without years of continued research, much of the anecdotal evidence is suggesting that an uncanny relationship may exist between the two components.

| "Could MS be a disease hinged on basic endocannabinoid deficiency? Anecdotal evidence on CBD use has suggested that an uncanny relationship may exist between the two components…"

For the time being, at least, it seems multiple sclerosis sufferers will continue to have to rely on self-treatment methods, and, unless they live in a medically legalized state, will have to resort to "non-conventional" approaches in order to obtain alternative medications like CBD oil.

The impossibly comical irony of the federal government owning a medically-viable patent to CBD, while maintaining a Schedule I status on the plant that it comes from, is a discussion that will have to wait for another time and another place.

Whatever means an MS sufferer might have to go to in order to receive treatment and receive the parts of their life back that the disease took from them, though, is a decidedly small price to pay in the grand scheme of things.

Current Research on Cannabis and Multiple Sclerosis

Believe it or not, dozens of academic and research publications have come out in recent years with regard to the use of cannabinoids as a potential MS treatment. Here, we point out five of the most relevant studies to date. But beware – the information contained herein may make you violently angry when considering the fact that the government has not pursued clinical trials for the use of CBD on multiple sclerosis.

The Role of CBD Products in Managing Multiple Sclerosis

Cannabidiol (CBD) is a non-psychoactive compound found in the cannabis plant often used by patients as an oil to manage the symptoms of chronic conditions.

According to the National Multiple Sclerosis Society, more than two million people have MS worldwide. Cannabidiol is a non-psychoactive compound found in the cannabis plant often used by patients as an oil to manage the symptoms of some chronic conditions.

Multiple sclerosis is a varied condition from individual to the next. Some of the things that we do see that are more common would be sensory symptoms – numbness and tingling. Unfortunately, some of these sensory symptoms can be quite painful, so there's not just plain old numbness, but there could be a burning sensation. Some of the other things that are common with multiple sclerosis would be increased muscle tone or spasming that can leave people with very painful cramping throughout the day and night. We see cognitive issues with multiple sclerosis – trouble with memory or with processing speed. One of the things that is more obvious to the public might be mobility issues, so people that need a cane, a walker, a wheelchair or a power chair to help get around within that umbrella of multiple sclerosis that we see so many varied patterns from one person to the next.

Q: We hear about the many medications that patients with MS are on, sometimes even cocktail, but it's getting much more advanced. Just generally, what are some of the typical medications or how many medications are they typically on to deal with some of these challenging symptoms?

ANS: Science has advanced rapidly in our ability to manage multiple sclerosis. We don't have a cure yet, but we are getting closer. We now have 16 FDA approved treatment options in the United States for alternating the long-term course of multiple sclerosis. One of the goals with MS would be to stop the progression in its track, to not let things advance any further. There are two other buckets of treatment that we see out there, and that would be symptom management – managing some of those things that I mentioned earlier, like spasticity and the burning hypersensitivity. The third bucket would be treating acute attacks, so if someone woke up with a new neurological symptom, we can use things like steroid medications to hopefully shorten the duration of those symptoms. The average person with multiple sclerosis is on about six different medications just for their MS, and that's not counting other health conditions. That can be both a blessing and a challenge in that we have to be cautious about using so many medications and then worrying about side effects of different drugs and drug interactions also.

Q: Tell us a little bit about Cannabidiol and this non-psychoactive compound found in the cannabis plant. How can it possibly help MS patients?

ANS: There's been a lot of interest in recent years in the broad class of chemicals called cannabinoids. Cannabinoids are some of the chemical ingredients in the cannabis plant. There are over 400 cannabinoids. The two that have been most focused on are cannabidiol, or CBD, and then THC. THC would be the psychoactive part that people are more familiar with. Cannabidiol, as you mentioned, is the non-psychoactive part of the plant. There is a quite a body of literature out there looking at the use of cannabinoids to manage certain multiple sclerosis symptoms. Most commonly, we think of CBD as being something that we might use in the management of spasticity or in the management of these painful areas of hypersensitivity in people with multiple sclerosis. When we talked about those three buckets of MS treatment, managing relapses, managing symptoms and then changing long-term course, we could typically think of CBD to fit in that second bucket, or managing symptoms.

Q: How is it administered? What's its effect on the body and is this a controversial type of thing to use?

ANS: The use of cannabinoids, the bigger class, can be a little bit controversial and also a little bit confusing. 43 states in the United States now have some sort of law in the book regarding the use of medical cannabis whether it's CBD or the whole plant material. Those laws vary from state to state, and many of those laws actually contradict what the federal law says. It leaves individuals very confused. It leaves healthcare providers very confused at times. CBA can be administered most commonly as an oil, which is taken by mouth. It would come in a small bottle and you would have something like a medicine dropper that looks like an eyedropper to put the medicine under the tongue. There are forms out there in a vaporizer so that you could put that into an inhaled form. There are edible forms as well, but most commonly, individuals with MS are used in an oil form through a medicine dropper.

Q: Is this something that now will go along with their medications or only used as needed for certain symptoms?

ANS: We think of CBD as fitting in for symptom management like for the spasticity or pain, and it could be either used on an ass needed basis or as a maintenance medication. The challenge for us right now is finding reliable sources for people to obtain the oil and then hopefully being able to partner with whoever is providing that oil to help guide individual with MS. Personally, what I would like to do, if I have an individual with MS who's already on some symptomatic medications, is add the oil to their existing regimen, see how they do with it and then hopefully be able to back off on some of their other prescription medications.

Q: I know this is based on upcoming studies, but do you see that it might have an effect on the long-term or is it simply palliative in nature?

ANS: There is a lot of interest out there in cannabinoids for the long-term management of MS, in other words, fitting into that third bucket. Can we actually change the course of MS and do more than just symptom management? The background for that is that humans do have something called the endocannabinoid system. We have chemicals in our body made naturally that look like some of these cannabinoids and they seem to function primarily in the central nervous, but interestingly also in the immune system. There is quite a bit of interest out there in potentially using cannabinoids to tone down the over-activity of multiple sclerosis. On paper, it looks very promising. To date, no one's been able to definitely show that, but it is certainly an area of quite a bit of interest.

Q: Does someone need a medical marijuana prescription to take CBD?

ANS: This again is where things get a little bit confusing. There is a federal law that was passed in 2014 called the CBD Oil Act that allowed for the production of CBD oil from hemp. Hemp is a subspecies of cannabis that produces very little THC. At least one federal law says that CBD can be purchased legally in all 50 states. In spite of that, CBD is still listed as a schedule one compound where we put it with heroin and cocaine and things like that, so this is sometimes where the laws are very contradictory. That said, there are a number of sites out there where you can purchase pure CBD oil without THC in it. It is a case of buyer beware, so the FDA has sent out some warning letters to manufacturers who probably were not producing legitimate CBD oil or maybe what they said was in the bottle was not actually in the bottle. Ideally, you'd like to see a laboratory certificate from the manufacturer that says that this is a reliable source of CBD. When you get into compounds with THC in it, that's where you're going to have to look at your state laws and see what the individual state says and how you would go about legally having access to that. For us here in Georgia, we have the low TBH CBD oil law saying that for 15 different health conditions, if you are registered with the state, you can possess CBD oil with up to 5% THC in it.

Q: Are there any side effects? Does it give a bit of a high as if you were using another one of the cannabinoids or is this something different?

ANS: Pure CBD oil is non-psychoactive, so people cannot get high from it. We do hear people sometimes say they have a calming effect with it, but nothing that would impair your cognition or driving ability. Once you get into compounds or oils where there is THC, then you do have to start looking at that potential that someone could actually have a euphoric effect or actually get high from it. We typically think of some of these cannabinoids as having an anti-nausea effect. Many of the states where there is some sort of cannabis legislation, they have seen an increase in people reporting this paradoxical increase in nausea, and that's usually a result of excessive THC use, so people ended up in the emergency room with cycles of nausea and vomiting because they're using too much of a

THC compound. The treatment for that is simply getting them on less THC or taking it away altogether.

Q: Wrap it up for us with your best advice and information on CBD products in managing multiple sclerosis, what you want people to know and what questions you would like them to ask their physician if they're somebody with MS and they're dealing with some of these symptoms that they're having trouble and challenging managing these symptoms, what you want them to ask about CBD.

ANS: I would advise people with multiple sclerosis to become knowledgeable about their individual state law, what is in the book, what are you allowed to have and then try to discuss that with their treating neurologist or healthcare team if you have symptoms of multiple sclerosis, like pain or spasticity, that might be amenable to treatment with a CBD product. Talk to your healthcare team, and at the same time, I would ask the patient with your healthcare team this whole area is evolving so rapidly, and for a lot of people, they didn't receive training in medical school or nursing school or PA school on cannabinoids and where they might fit into the use in multiple sclerosis or other health conditions. I would say know your local laws, look at your resources that are out there, try to partner with your healthcare team, and then if you do end up using a CBD or CBD THC product, do your homework. Make sure that you're getting that from a reliable source. If possible, you want to see a laboratory certificate to show that this is what you think it is.

Effects of Cannabinoids and CBD on Multiple Sclerosis

Research findings suggest that cannabis could slow the neurodegenerative process of multiple sclerosis. Studies have shown that cannabinoids are involved in the regulation of the immune system by way of acting upon the cannabinoid receptors of the endocannabinoid system. Cannabinoids have shown they can modulate the inflammatory reaction and assist in neuroregeneration2,6. In one study, cannabinoids demonstrated neuroprotective effects during an animal model of multiple sclerosis, reducing the damage to myelin caused from inflammation10. Another study found that cannabinoids administered to animals with a model of multiple sclerosis reduced neurological disability, improved motor coordination and limited the progression of the disease.

Cannabis can help multiple sclerosis patients manage the symptoms associated with their disease. Cannabis has shown to be effective at reducing pain, muscle stiffness and spasms in multiple sclerosis patients5,12. In one study, multiple sclerosis patients saw significant improvements in muscle spasticity and reduced sleep disturbances after four weeks of cannabis treatment8. A similar study found that multiple sclerosis patients experienced pain and sleep improvements after five weeks of treatment with cannabis containing both tetrahydrocannabinol (THC) and cannabidiol (CBD)11. In a questionnaire survey, multiple sclerosis patients responded that cannabis was effective in improving spasticity, chronic pain of extremities, tremors, emotional dysfunctions, fatigue, double vision, bowel and bladder dysfunctions, dysfunctions of walking and balance and memory loss.

There is some evidence that suggests that cannabis may worsen cognitive problems in multiple sclerosis patients. Multiple sclerosis patients that were regular users of street cannabis have scored significantly worse on cognitive function tests.

States That Have Approved Medical Cannabis for Multiple Sclerosis

Currently, 16 states have approved medical cannabis specifically for the treatment of multiple sclerosis. These states include Alaska, Connecticut, Florida, Georgia, Illinois, Louisiana, Maine, Massachusetts, New Hampshire, New Jersey, New Mexico, New York, Ohio, Pennsylvania, Vermont, and West Virginia. In Washington D.C., any condition can be approved for medical cannabis as long as a DC-licensed physician recommends the treatment.

A number of other states will consider allowing medical cannabis to be used for the treatment of multiple sclerosis with the recommendation from a physician. These states include: California (any debilitating illness where the medical use of cannabis has been recommended by a physician), Nevada (other conditions subject to approval), Oregon (other conditions subject to approval), Rhode Island (other conditions subject to approval), and Washington (any "terminal or debilitating condition").

Several states have approved medical cannabis specifically to treat "chronic pain," which is a symptom commonly associated with multiple sclerosis. These states include: Alaska, Arizona, California, Colorado, Delaware, Hawaii, Maine, Maryland, Michigan, Montana, New Mexico, Ohio, Oregon, Pennsylvania, Rhode Island, Vermont, and West Virginia. The states of Montana, Nevada, New Hampshire, North Dakota, Ohio, and Vermont allow medical cannabis to treat "severe pain." The states of Arkansas, Minnesota, Ohio, Pennsylvania, Washington, and West Virginia have approved cannabis for the treatment of "intractable pain."

Several states will allow medical cannabis for the treatment of spasms, which can arise in those with multiple sclerosis. These states include: Arizona, Arkansas, California, Colorado, Delaware, Florida, Hawaii, Louisiana,

Maryland, Michigan, Minnesota, Montana, Nevada, Oregon, Rhode Island, and Washington.

Patients whose multiple sclerosis causes seizures can use medical cannabis to treat that specific symptom in several states, including Alaska, Arizona, Arkansas, California, Colorado, Delaware, Florida, Hawaii, Louisiana, Maryland, Michigan, Minnesota, Montana, Nevada, New Hampshire, North Dakota, Ohio, Oregon, Pennsylvania (intractable seizures), Rhode Island, Tennessee (intractable seizures), Vermont, and Washington.

Recent Studies on Cannabinoids and CBD's Effect on Multiple Sclerosis

Cannabinoids were effective at reducing neurological disability and the progression of the disease in mice with an animal form of MS.

Cannabinoids ameliorate disease progression in a model of multiple sclerosis in mice, acting preferentially through CB1 receptor-mediated anti-inflammatory effects.

Four weeks of cannabis treatment caused significant spasm improvements in MS patients.

A randomized double-blind-placebo-controlled, parallel-group, enriched-design study of nabiximols* (Sativex(®), as add-on therapy, in subjects with refractory spasticity caused by multiple sclerosis

Five weeks of cannabis treatment significantly reduced pain and improved sleep in MS patients.

Randomized, controlled trial of cannabis-based medicine in central pain in multiple sclerosis.

CBD From Hemp and How It's Helped My MS

Over my time battling Multiple Sclerosis, there have been a few moments where I could point to something and say, wow, that's been extremely helpful and life-changing for me. Starting my current disease modifying therapy (DMT) has been certainly been one, in that it has slowed my progression when other DMTs couldn't. We don't take DMTs for our everyday symptoms though, so it's hard to realize their importance when we are still falling down, fatigued, or in pain. When it comes to my everyday symptoms, I've mentioned before how medical marijuana has been a game changer for me. Today, I want to discuss something related, but more accessible, to medical marijuana that has made a major impact on my life: CBD (cannabidiol) derived from Hemp.

Hemp vs. marijuana

As I explained in my medical marijuana article, the compounds that are most helpful for our symptoms are called cannabinoids. Cannabinoids mimic naturally occurring compounds in our body called endocannabinoids. The most basic description of how all this works is that these compounds can change and improve the way our cells communicate with each other. When we take in cannabinoids, they interact with the already existing endocannabinoid system of our bodies and the cannabinoid receptors found in all human cells. It's important to realize that these compounds are already part of us, and although these cannabinoids are coming from plants, they are still similar to the ones in our bodies.

When we talk about marijuana, the two cannabinoids we get the most of are CBD and THC. THC is the compound associated with the more psychoactive effects of marijuana. These effects can be very helpful to those with MS, however, they are also the reason marijuana is constantly fighting a legal battle. THC is what we associate with people getting "high". Most folks using medical marijuana will actually choose a strain that is higher in CBD than THC because it's the CBD cannabinoid that is often most effective in helping our symptoms like pain and spasms. Here is where hemp comes in! The hemp plant contains a good percentage of the CBD cannabinoid and a very low percentage of THC. So people can't really use it to get "high", but they can use it to extract CBD for its medicinal properties. Because of this, it is much easier to obtain CBD oil produced from hemp than from the cannabis plant.

Quality issues

This sounds great, right? It does, but the problem is that it isn't regulated. Producing and selling CBD oil has become a big business, but it can be extremely hard to find consistent and effective product. There are various extraction methods for getting CBD oil from the hemp plant, some more effective than others, and you rarely know which method a company has used. That can making finding a consistent and effective CBD product difficult. It can also mean that many will try CBD oil and not have a positive experience and think it simply won't work for them, when in reality, they just acquired a batch that was poorly extracted.

My experience

I'm most certainly not an expert on all things CBD, but I did do some research and found a place online that seemed well-reviewed and looked like they knew what they were doing. I was still very skeptical, more so than I was with medical marijuana. I purchased a bottle of CBD tincture that contained 500 mg of CBD into a 2 ounce bottle. I then began using this tincture each day by placing a few drops under my tongue. I found that the key for me was doing this every day regardless of how bad my symptoms were. For me, it is not an instant helper, in fact, if I know I will be extra busy on a Tuesday, I'll take extra on that Monday. Consistency has been the important factor to me. When I take it every day, or even close to every day, my body is much better off. Less pain, less spasticity, and less fatigue. Hard to believe, even for me. This is one of the few things I've taken where I've had multiple people come up and asked me if anything changed, because they can see that I am out more and I am more active. I've been using this for close to eight months now and I can honestly say it's made a huge difference in my life.

I know not everyone will have the same experience as me (remember, we're all a little different), but I wanted to share what it's done for me. I stress that consistency and quality are important aspects of CBD usage for me. Quality CBD products can be expensive, though in my experience, less expensive than medical marijuana and much more easily obtainable (you do not need a special medical marijuana card or prescription). If you have the means and desire, go ahead and try it. As always, do some research on your own as well, there is a wealth of resources and groups related to CBD use for chronic illness.

I Tried Hemp Oil for My MS, and Here's What Happened

I've had multiple sclerosis (MS) for almost a decade, and while I'm on what's considered to be the most powerful, last attempt, treatment ... most of my decade of MS has been about trying anything that might work.

Once I was diagnosed, I immediately became a juicer. I juice as many greens a day, as possible. I stopped consuming dairy, gluten, yeast, wheat, most oats, sugar, caffeine, and anything else one might find in a grocery. Kidding. Sort of.

I rely heavily on chiropractic care and medications. And, yet, the one, almost laughable thing I didn't know about was hemp oil. When my friend told me she was a representative for a hemp oil company, and thought it would be helpful for my peripheral neuropathy at night, I just stood there with my mouth open. I had no idea about what it was or how it differed from medical marijuana, even.

So I did what I always do. I texted my doctor. His response?: "Go for it!"

So, what's hemp

Hemp is a really tall plant with big, thick stalk that grows to about 15 feet tall. That's huge compared to marijuana, which barely clears five feet. They grow in varying ways and different parts are important to different people, for a variety of reasons.

Hemp is both legal and considered safe, hence my doctor's response. Because of that, it's reported to be grown in over 30 different countries. Because medical marijuana isn't legal everywhere in the United States, and controversial all over the world, we don't have an accurate report of where it's grown.

What makes these plants of interest to scientists, healers, and those in need of treatment is cannabidiol, or CBD. CBD is present in both hemp and marijuana, but what makes marijuana psychoactive — giving you the 'high' sensation — is tetrahydrocannabinol (THC). Hemp contains only trace amounts of THC, and studies have shown that CBD is not psychoactive like THC.

The way I explain it to anyone now is: Hemp doesn't go high. It hits low. It's considered to be soothing and relaxing.

Strategies to Fine-Tune Your CBD Oil Dosage

By and large, the acceptance and use of cannabidiol as a therapeutic, healing substance is in its infancy. Medical professionals and scientists are only now beginning to develop dosing schedules for medical marijuana, medicinal hemp, and their extracts (including CBD).

Even with the current wave of states legalizing medical marijuana, many physicians are hesitant to prescribe cannabinoids like CBD. This is for two reasons:

1 – Doctors cannot prescribe (only recommend) cannabinoids, because there's no recommended daily allowance (RDA) or universal dose for all people.

2 – Most medical schools never cover CBD/cannabidiol therapy in their pharmacology courses (the drug curriculum revolves primarily around substances that can be patented).

Because there is no recommended dose, the information presented on this page is intended to serve only as an informational guide – a starting point of reference – and should never be considered medical advice.

When it comes to cannabinoids, there is one universal truth to keep in mind:

Everyone Is Different

There are countless variables such as weight, diet, metabolism, genetics, environment, product consistency, and more that make a universally prescribed dosage an impossibility.

While we wish we could provide the public with a mathematical CBD dosage calculator, it isn't quite that simple – very rough estimates are about as good as it gets.

With these facts in mind, most people who are new to cannabidiol begin their journey by starting with the minimal suggested CBD dosage on any product, then gradually increasing the dose until they achieve the desired results.

The (COR) Serving Standard is 25mg of CBD, taken twice daily.

Additionally, our analysis suggests increasing the amount of CBD you take every 3-4 weeks by 25mg until you attain symptom relief (inversely, decrease by 25mg if symptoms worsen).

Additionally, you might find it useful to record your daily experiences in a notebook so you can accurately narrow in on what works and feels best for you. With that understanding in place, it is now time to learn more about CBD oil and how to find the right CBD oil dosage for you.

How Much CBD Oil Should I Take

Mayo Clinic suggests CBD dosages based on scientific research, publications, traditional use, and expert opinion. Cannabinoid dosages and duration of treatment depend mainly on the illness (and countless other factors).

- Loss of Appetite in Cancer Patients: 2.5mg of THC (orally), with or without 1mg of CBD for six weeks. [S]
- Chronic Pain: 2.5-20mg of CBD [with or without THC] (orally). [S]
- Epilepsy: 200-300mg of CBD (orally) daily. [S]
- Movement Problems Due to Huntington's Disease: 10mg of CBD per kg of body weight daily for six weeks (orally). [S]
- Sleep Disorders: 40mg-160mg of CBD (orally). [S]
- Multiple Sclerosis (MS) symptoms: Cannabis plant extracts containing 2.5-120 milligrams of a THC/CBD combination daily for 2-15 weeks. Patients typically use eight sprays within any three hours, with a maximum of 48 sprays in any 24-hour period. [S]
- Schizophrenia: 40-1,280mg oral CBD daily. [S]

- Glaucoma: A single sublingual CBD dosage of 20-40mg (>40 mg may increase eye pressure). [S]

Learn the Types of CBD Products

CBD hemp oil comes in seemingly endless forms, each with a different concentration of CBD and other phytocannabinoids. Determining how to use CBD oil first starts with choosing your route of administration – in other words, choosing the best way to take CBD oil for your needs and lifestyle.

These include…

Ingestibles:

- Liquid hemp oil, like CBD tinctures or CBD drops
- CBD concentrated into a thick paste (often referred to as Rick Simpson Oil, or RSO)
- Encapsulated CBD oil
- Phytocannabinoid-rich sprays/spritzers (generally designed for application beneath the tongue)
- Bottled water containing nano-sized CBD particles
- CBD-infused chewing gum
- On-the-go dissolvable powders containing CBD (oftentimes blended with other adaptogenic herbs)
- Cooking oils (such as coconut oil or olive oil) with added cannabinoids

- CBD-infused edibles (i.e., gummies, brownies, cookies, etc.; generally for individuals who are sensitive to smoking/vaping)

Smokables:

- Crystalline isolates
- Wax (similar to THC-containing marijuana concentrates called "shatter")
- CBD-rich eLiquids and/or vape cartridges (akin to an e-cigarette)

Topicals:

- Transdermal patches with CBD (similar to a nicotine patch)
- Cannabidiol-infused salves,balms, lotions, shampoos, or soaps (for topical use)
- Bath bombs infused with CBD
- Decide How to Use CBD Oil

While many options like chewing gum need no instructions, we have compiled these tips on how to take CBD oil:

- Liquid CBD Oil/Tinctures/Extracts: Drops or tinctures should have a "suggested serving size" and the total milligrams of CBD listed on their packaging. From there, you can determine the amount of CBD you would like to ingest. Simply place the correct quantity of drops under your tongue using the dropper and hold the CBD oil in place for a minimum of 60 seconds. The 60 second hold allows for absorption via the blood vessels underneath your tongue efficiently bypassing first-pass metabolism. Once 60 seconds has passed, swallow the CBD oil.

- CBD E-Liquid/Vape Cartridges: Vaping is excellent for people looking for an immediate response, as inhalation is the fastest way to deliver CBDs to your brain and body. To use vape simply exhale gently the air from your lungs then inhale through the mouthpiece slowly for 3 seconds. Then fill your lungs the rest of the way with additional breath and hold for a few seconds, exhaling when ready. There are pre-filled, cost-effective vape pens and cartridges available as well as more expensive vaporizers that you can refill with CBD-infused e-liquid.

- CBD Edibles: With edibles, the only required steps are open, eat, and enjoy! This method of consumption will result in more drawn-out effects that also take longer to kick in than some of the other options. Edibles are great for those seeking sustained effects, or for those who want to be subtle about their usage of CBDs.

- CBD Isolates/Concentrates: Anyone familiar with smoking hash or other cannabis concentrates like wax and BHO will be no stranger to this delivery method. Simply sprinkle some into a vaporizer or water pipe, ignite, inhale, and enjoy! We find that this option is useful for individuals looking to elevate their regular consumption of CBD-rich cannabis flowers or other smokable herbs.

Choose a CBD Brand with a Dosage You Can Trust

Figuring out how much CBD oil to take can feel like trying to navigate through a complicated maze. The sheer volume of CBD brands on the market can create confusion for consumers, and when you take a closer look, it's not difficult to understand why. Not only do vendors use different source materials (CBD-rich cannabis vs. industrial hemp, different strains, etc.), but they also implement different extraction techniques .

Adding to the confusion, many vendors recommend excessive doses, while others suggest amounts that are a fraction of what experts would consider effective.

As with a fermented food like kombucha, slight natural variations are normal and to be expected in a product such as CBD oil because it is made from living plants. Changes in the weather, soil, and water can all impact the biology of the source material. While we verify Certificates of Analysis (and take many other criteria into consideration during our review process), even the most reputable five-star companies have no way to control for every variable in this organic process.

While perhaps not as ideal as a CBD dosage chart, we at CBD Oil Review (COR) have created an official COR Serving Standard through an extensive analysis of hundreds of products.

The (COR) Serving Standard is 25mg of CBD, taken twice daily.

Additionally, our analysis suggests increasing the amount of CBD you take every 3-4 weeks by 25mg until you attain symptom relief (inversely, decrease by 25mg if symptoms worsen).

Consider Why Your Health Would Benefit from CBD

Cannabinoids such as CBD have a dizzying array of functions in the human body, influencing everything from inflammation to anxiety and depression. You don't necessarily need to have a serious illness to benefit from

CBD; even healthy individuals can experience a remarkable increase in their quality of life with its use.

The following is a chart of illnesses/conditions that whose symptoms may be relieved by CBD:

- Pain (neuropathic, chronic etc.)
- Epilepsy
- Multiple Sclerosis (MS)
- Amyotrophic Lateral Sclerosis (ALS)
- Parkinson's
- Inflammation
- Acne
- Dyskinesia
- Psoriasis
- Broken Bones
- Mad Cow Disease
- Depression
- Bacterial Infections
- Diabetes
- Rheumatoid Arthritis
- Nausea
- Anxiety
- ADHD
- Schizophrenia
- Substance Abuse/Withdrawal
- Heart Disease

- Irritable Bowel Syndrome (IBS)

Keep in mind that this CBD benefits list is in no way complete; we are only beginning to discover how cannabinoids can help.

Know You Cannot Overdose on CBD

There is no established lethal dose of CBD, and chronic use/high doses of up to 1500 mg per day (30x MORE than the COR Serving Standard!) have been repeatedly shown to be well tolerated by humans.

As with any natural product, it is important to speak with your physician prior to beginning use. There are some slight risks associated with using CBD in high doses or for extended periods of time, including:

- Mild Low Blood Pressure
- Dry Mouth
- Lightheadedness
- Sedation
- Reduced activity of T and B Cells
- Decreased Fertilization Capacity
- Reduced p-Glycoprotein activity
- Reduced activity of Cytochrome P450 (CYP450) Enzyme

Keep in mind that these side effects illustrate worst-case scenarios with CBD, and are not necessarily typical.

There is one major exception to the "generally harmless" attitude about CBD and that is the negative effect cannabinoids can have on the functioning of the liver's CYP450 enzyme. Approximately 60% of all pharmaceutical drugs undergo metabolism by this enzyme, including:

- Steroids
- HMG CoA reductase inhibitors
- Calcium channel blockers
- Antihistamines
- Prokinetics
- HIV-antivirals
- Immune modulators
- Benzodiazepines
- Antiarrhythmics
- Antibiotics
- Anesthetics
- Antipsychotics
- Antidepressants
- Anti-epileptics
- Beta blockers
- PPIs
- NSAIDs
- Angiotensin II blockers
- Oral hypoglycemic agents

- Sulfonylureas

Before you start taking CBD, please read about drug interactions.

It is important to note that even something as benign as grapefruit juice can cause the same CYP450 enzyme inhibitory action as CBD.

The most important things to do before taking CBD (or any other herbal product) are research any possible drug interactions and talk with your physician to address any additional questions regarding CBD drug interactions or overdose concerns. You and your doctor together will always know best!

Understand How Your Genetics Impact CBD Dosing

As if you didn't have enough factors to consider when deciding your ideal CBD oil dosage, now you have to think about how your own genetics can impact this amount.

Some individuals have been found to have mutations on the CNR1 gene, which is responsible for coding the CB1 receptor (a type of receptor in cells throughout your body that interacts with cannabinoids). Issues with the CNR1 gene can ultimately result in a poorly functioning endocannabinoid system, which is an important variable when figuring out how to use CBD oil.

Here are some other cellular-level factors that can affect how CBD is absorbed in your body:

- Various substances can profoundly affect CB1 receptors. Certain lifestyle choices can impact how your body metabolizes CBD.

What does this mean? Well, for example, THC increases the activity of CB1 receptors, while ethanol (alcohol) increases its expression. So, theoretically, smoking cannabis and drinking alcohol may increase the effects of CBD.

- Morphine and epinephrine decrease the activity of the CB1 receptor.

What does this mean? It may mean those currently using opiates could, with approval and guidance from their physician, find CBD useful in decreasing opiate use .

- Exercise and nicotine both increase anandamide levels (while similar to THC – this is a cannabinoid that we naturally synthesize in our brains) which is a natural CB1 receptor activator.

What does this mean? Being active, as well as ingesting nicotine (while the latter is not recommended), might increase the effects of CBD.

- DHA (an omega-3 fatty acid) increases CB1 receptors.

What does this mean? Theoretically, those eating a diet rich in fatty fish would naturally need to use less CBD oil.

- Prolonged elevated glucocorticoids (such as cortisol) reduce CB1 receptor density.

What does this mean? Those under high levels of chronic stress would potentially need higher CBD oil dosage to achieve the same effects achieved by people who are not chronically stressed.

We are only beginning to understand genetics, and as such it's a good idea to take anything related to this emerging science with a grain of salt. As with any natural substance, consult with your physician about any questions and/or concerns you may have regarding CBD and how to use CBD oil.

Rest Easy Knowing CBD Oil Is Not Physically Addictive

People often ask us, "Can I get addicted to CBD oil?" This is a tricky question, and the answer ultimately depends on your school of thought.

Based strictly on chemistry, the answer is no. Cannabidiol is not physically addictive in the same way substances like heroin, cocaine, alcohol, opiates, benzodiazepines, and related substances can be. Further, CBD cannot produce any physical withdrawal symptoms in and of itself upon cessation of use.

(Interestingly, CBD is currently undergoing study for its ability to minimize withdrawal from drugs with severe cessation symptoms, like opiates.)

However, human beings can get addicted to just about anything that isn't chemically addicting: exercise, music, sex, and food are great examples.

Those who take CBD daily to relieve symptoms of chronic illness and other severe conditions may find that their unpleasant sensations return shortly after they miss a dose. This is no different than one's headache returning once the effects of ibuprofen wear off.

However, because CBD can alter the levels of essential liver enzymes, it is crucial to do your research, talk to your physician, and figure out the best way to take CBD oil for your specific situation. Information and education will be your allies in your quest for healing.

Get the Most Bang for Your Buck

If you've been using CBD products for some time without verifying the potency through their vendors, it's highly probable you've been using a minimally effective formulation that hasn't been delivering as much CBD as you thought (or as much as you've paid for!).

This is why CBD Oil Review exists, why we've created our five-badge rating system, and why we've enlisted independent reviewers to verify that CBD companies are being ethical.

Most doctors don't specialize medicinal cannabis and CBD oil. This means they may not be able to help you as thoroughly as you had hoped and they may be unable to offer guidance when it comes to helping you decide how much CBD oil to take. It is also worth noting that many patients feel uncomfortable talking to their doctor about cannabis and CBD.

If you have detailed questions about how much CBD oil to take, how to take CBD oil, drug interactions, or just want to know what to do next, consult with a cannabis doctor today!

Why is it so fascinating to the world of neurological disorders

CBD has been shown to have significant antioxidant and neuroprotective properties, suggesting that it could be a potential treatment for neurological disorders.

While CBD is not yet FDA-approved for any condition, many studies and user testimonies have shown promising results for a variety of indications.

I used to treat a student with a very aggressive seizure disorder. It was so aggressive, I couldn't turn the lights on or off in our room while she was there or it could trigger a grand mal seizure. I was talking to her mother on the phone about her progress one day and she confided in me that she'd started using hemp oil, rubbing it on her daughter at night, and that she hadn't had a seizure since. I was happy to hear.

Overcoming the stigma

I think there's a stigma attached to hemp products, which is why her mother told me in confidence. It's also why I didn't find out about how many people use it for multiple conditions until I began to try it for my own peripheral neuropathy and spasticity.

People are scared they'll be judged. It's not medical marijuana though I don't believe anyone should be judged for their personal treatment plans if it involves this, either. It's both safe and legal, without psychoactive effects.

So, I began to use the oil on my feet and lower legs, massaging it on topically at night. I almost feel bad saying this I haven't had one bad night, in terms of peripheral neuropathy and spasticity in my lower limbs, since trying the Ananda hemp oil.

But it was a different story with the pill form, which I was told would relax me before bed. One study showed that hemp seed supplements with other oils had beneficial effects of improving symptoms in people with MS. But my experience was so bad, I don't want to rehash.

We believe we had the dosage wrong we were way off, in my humble opinion and my friend has begged me to try it again. But for now, I'm too afraid. And frankly, I don't feel that I need it.

I get so much relief from the topical form, I can't even put it into words. That is all I wanted. I never dreamed anything would work this well.

Bottom line

So should you run out and get hemp oil from the health aisle in the grocery store? No, it's not that simple. Not all hemp oil is created equal.

There are certifications and regulations that testify to the quality of the hemp used. These certifications are important because they're essentially the brand's credentials. You must research the brand you use. I chose Ananda hemp because they had every certification possible, and they're affiliated with a higher learning institution to do further research.

Hemp oil isn't for everyone. How effective it is will depend on your individual symptoms, biology, and dosage. And research hasn't yet proven its effectiveness. But it's worked for me, and may work for you.

My advice is to not walk into the world of hemp oil blindly. Discuss your treatment options with your doctor and do thorough research on the different brands and forms of hemp oil before you take the leap.

Best CBD Oils for Multiple Sclerosis

As it turns out, not all CBD oils are exactly the same. While they all, of course, rely on cannabidiol as the active component, some specific tinctures have shown to be far more effective at treating symptoms stemming from MS than have others.

While a full-spectrum cannabis CBD oil is thought to be the best option, these oils are often not available nationwide. With that said, there are a few companies that seem to be helping with various symptoms associated with multiple sclerosis. Here are our top 5 favorite ones [with two extras that we had to throw in as "honorable mentions!"]:

Made in the USA
Middletown, DE
14 July 2020